I0791570

ISBN: 9781650802695

7-DAY

VEGETARIAN DIET
PESCETARIAN

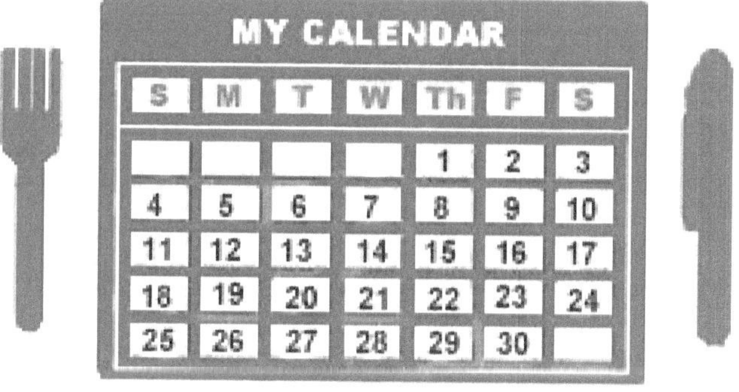

S. Vjay Gupta
Gail Johnson, M.S.

NoPaperPress™

CONTENTS

The 90-Day Vegetarian Diet blends American cooking with Asian vegetarian concepts. Of course this diet is meatless, but fish, eggs and dairy are allowed. The diet is a Pescetarian version of vegetarianism and features delicious, low calorie, nutritionally balanced vegetarian meals.

A well planned vegetarian diet can provide the same level of nutrients as a meat-eater's diet. In addition, eating meat-free can have real weight-loss benefits because plant-based foods, such as vegetables, beans and whole grains, are loaded with fiber that help you feel satisfied on fewer calories. And many health-care professionals also think that eating a healthy vegetarian diet is one of the best things you can do for your short-term and long-term health.

With this eBook, NoPaperPress publishes a popular vegetarian variant: the **Pesceterian Vegetarian Diet** that includes fish, eggs and dairy products. And all NoPaperPress vegetarian diet eBooks come in 90-day, 30-day and 7-day editions. For background and nutritional information and more on vegetarianism see Appendix A (page 34).

When to Use the 7-Day Diet

If you're in weight maintenance mode but notice your weight creeping up. You want to stop the upward trend and lose a few pounds as well. Here's the perfect solution: Use the *7-Day Vegetarian Diet* to quickly lose those unwanted few pounds!

You've let your weight get out of control. So you decide to go on a diet. It doesn't matter what diet, or how much weight you want to lose. Your first move should be to go on the *7-Day Diet* lose a quick 3 to 5 pounds and get on the right track. After the 7-day diet does its job you can switch to a longer-term diet. My suggestion would be either the 30-Day Vegetarian Diet or the 90-Day Vegetarian Diet, both eBooks published by NoPaperPress.

Additionally, before you begin any weight loss program you need to make sure your health will allow you to lower your caloric intake and increase your physical activity. A **medical checkup** is in order which may be as simple as a visit to a physician who is familiar with your medical history, or it may be a thorough physical exam. The physician conducting the medical exam should be made aware of and should approve the specific weight loss diet you're planning

What's in this eBook?

This eBook actually contains two 7-day diets: a 1,200 Calorie diet, and for even faster weight loss a 900 Calorie diet. Both diets have a meal plan (menu) for each of the seven days. And every day features a "Recipe and Diet Tip of the Day."

Which Calorie Level is for You?

900 Calorie Diet: Smaller women, older women and inactive women should select the 900 Calorie diet.

1,200 Calorie Diet: Larger women, younger women and active women should choose the 1,200 Calorie diet. In the short term this is a good diet for all healthy men.

Note: Due to the very low calorie level, the 900-Calorie diet may not quite provide the protein, carbs, fat, vitamins, minerals and fiber you need for good health. Since it's a short term (7-Day) diet, however, this should not be a problem for most healthy people. If you have any health problems or concerns, you definitely should avoid the 900-Calorie diet. Additionally, because nearly everyone feels hungry on 900 Calories per day, this is not an easy diet to stay with.

How Much Weight Will You Lose?

Weight loss occurs when your food energy intake is less than the total energy you expend. This difference in calories is referred to as your <u>calorie deficit</u>. How much weight you lose depends on the magnitude of your calorie deficit. Physiologists have long known that to lose one pound requires a deficit of approximately 3,500 Calories. Therefore, if a person's total calorie deficit over time is known, their weight loss over time can be calculated.

On the 7-Day Diet, **most women lose 3 to 4 pounds** – depending on whether they select the 1,200 or 900 Calorie diet. Smaller women, older women and less active women will lose a bit less and larger women, younger women and more active women somewhat more.

On the 7-Day Diet, **most men lose 4 to 5 pounds** on the 1,200 diet. Smaller men, older men and less active men will lose a bit less and larger men, younger men and more active men quite a bit more.

Exactly how much weight you will lose depends on how much you weigh, your age and your activity level.For the full story see *Weight Control - U.S. Edition* by Vincent Antonetti, Ph.D, also published by NoPaperPress.

How to Use This eBook

First, depending on your size, your age and how active you are, choose the diet calorie level that's right for you, either 900 or 1,200 Calories per day.

   - **900-Calorie Diet go to page 9.**
   - **1200-Calorie Diet go to page 17.**

900 Calorie Meal Plans

Day 1 – 900 Calorie Meal Plan

BREAKFAST	Calories	Totals
Orange juice (½ cup)	50	
Wheaties (¾ cup) + ½ cup skim milk + ½ banana	190	
Coffee (Notes - page 42)	10	250 Cal
SNACK		
Coffee or tea	10	10 Cal
LUNCH		
Soup (Appendix C - page 42)	130	
Lettuce & tomato sandwich (1 Tbsp light mayo)	150	
Hot or iced tea	10	290 Cal
SNACK		
Coffee or tea	10	10 Cal
DINNER		
Baked salmon w salsa (Day 1 Recipe - page 25)	215	
Summer squash, zucchini and tomatoes	60	
Tossed green salad w 1½ Tbsp low-cal dressing*	70	
Water	0	345 Cal
* See page 40.		
SNACK		
Coffee or tea	10	10 Cal
		915 Cal

Day 2 – 900 Calorie Meal Plan

BREAKFAST	Calories	Totals
Orange juice (½ cup)	50	
Soft-boiled egg (**Notes** - page 41)	80	
Whole-grain toast (1 slice) (page 40)	65	
Coffee	10	205 Cal
SNACK		
Coffee or tea	10	10 Cal
LUNCH		
Salad (3 oz tuna, 1 tsp Evoo, onions & celery)	175	
Lettuce & tomato wedges	20	
Rye bread (1 slice)	65	
Diet soda or water	0	290 Cal
SNACK		
Coffee or tea	10	10 Cal
DINNER		
Portobello burger (**Day 2 Recipe**- page 26)	100	
Whole-grain roll (medium)	140	
Large tossed green salad w 1½ Tbsp low-cal dressing	70	
Fresh fruit in season (apple, peach, etc)	70	
Waterefw	0	380 Cal
SNACK		
Coffee or tea	10	10 Cal
		905 Cal

Day 3 – 900 Calorie Meal Plan

BREAKFAST	Calories	Totals
Tomato juice (½ cup)	20	
Two blueberry pancakes (Day 3a Recipe - p.27)	190	
Light syrup* (1 Tbsp)	30	
Coffee	10	250 Cal
*Max of 30 Cal per Tbsp.		
SNACK		
Coffee or tea	10	10 Cal
LUNCH		
Peanut butter (1 Tbsp) on 1 slice bread	170	
Skim milk (4 oz)	45	
Fresh fruit in season (peach, pear, etc)	70	285 Cal
SNACK		
Coffee or tea	10	10 Cal
DINNER		
Eggplant Parmesan (Day 3b Recipe- page 28)	270	
Large tossed green salad with 1½ Tbsp low-cal	70	
Water	0	340 Cal
SNACK		
Coffee or tea	10	10 Cal
		905 Cal

Day 4 – 900 Calorie Meal Plan

BREAKFAST	Calories	Totals
Orange juice (½ cup)	50	
Cheerios (1 cup) + ½ cup skim milk	160	
Coffee	10	220 Cal
SNACK		
Coffee or tea	10	10 Cal
LUNCH		
Cottage cheese (1 cup low fat)	180	
Large tossed green salad with 1½ Tbsp low-cal	70	
Water	0	250 Cal
SNACK		
Handful unsalted mixed nuts	100	100 Cal
DINNER		
Tofu Veggie Stir Fry (Day 4 Recipe - page 29)	230	
Fresh fruit in season (apple, pear, etc)	70	
Water	0	300 Cal
SNACK		
Coffee or tea	10	10 Cal
		890 Cal

Day 5 – 900 Calorie Meal Plan

BREAKFAST	Calories	Totals
Orange juice (½ cup)	50	
Wheaties (¾ cup) + ½ cup skim milk + ½ banana	190	
Coffee	10	250 Cal
SNACK		
Coffee or tea	10	10 Cal
LUNCH		
Grilled Swiss cheese sandwich (2 oz low-fat cheese)	310	
Pickle spear	0	
Diet soda or water	0	310 Cal
SNACK		
Coffee or tea	10	10 Cal
DINNER		
Frozen vegetarian entree (Day 5 Recipe page 30)	240	
Large tossed green salad w 1½ Tbsp low-cal dressing	70	
Water	0	310 Cal
SNACK		
Coffee or tea	10	10 Cal
		900 Cal

Day 6 – 900 Calorie Meal Plan

BREAKFAST	Calories	Totals
Orange juice (½ cup)	50	
Scrambled egg (Notes - page 42)	80	
Whole-grain toast (1 slice)	70	
Coffee	10	210 Cal
SNACK		
Coffee or tea	10	10 Cal
LUNCH		
Soup #8 (Appendix C - page 42)	160	
Tomato slices, ¼ cup chopped fresh basil + ½ tsp	40	
Whole-grain bread (1 slice)	70	270 Cal
SNACK		
Yogurt (6 oz, nonfat, any flavor)	90	90 Cal
DINNER		
Baked Herb-Crusted Cod (Day 6 Recipe page 31)	230	
Asparagus (7 spears cooked & drained)	20	
Fresh fruit in season (apple, plum, etc)	70	
Water		320 Cal
SNACK		
Coffee or tea	10	10 Cal
		905 Cal

Day 7 – 900 Calorie Meal Plan

BREAKFAST	Calories	Totals
Orange juice (½ cup)	50	
Cheerios (1 cup) + ½ cup milk* + about 15 raisins	190	
Coffee	10	250 Cal
* Always use skim milk in cereal.		
SNACK		
Coffee or tea	10	10 Cal
LUNCH		
Egg salad (1 egg + 1 Tbsp light mayo)	125	
Whole-grain bread (1 slice)	70	
Hot or iced tea	10	205 Cal
SNACK		
Coffee or tea	10	10 Cal
DINNER		
Pasta w Marinara sauce (Day 7 Recipe page 32)	225	
Large tossed green salad w 1½ Tbsp low-cal dressing	70	
Fresh fruit in season (peach, plum, etc)	70	
Water	0	365 Cal
SNACK		
Graham cracker (2 squares)	60	
Coffee or tea	10	70 Cal
		910 Cal

1200 Calorie Meal Plans

Day 1 – 1200 Calorie Meal Plan

BREAKFAST	Calories	Totals
Cantaloupe (½ medium)	50	
Wheaties (¾ cup) + ½ cup skim milk + ½ banana	190	
Coffee (Notes - page 42)	10	250 Cal
SNACK		
Coffee or tea	10	10 Cal
LUNCH		
Soup (Appendix C - page 42)	140	
Turkey breast (1 oz) on 1 slice rye breadandwich)	115	
Pickle spear	0	
Lettuce & tomato slices	20	
Hot or iced tea	10	285 Cal
SNACK		
Coffee or tea	10	10 Cal
DINNER		
Baked salmon w salsa (Day 1 Recipe - page 25)	215	
Summer squash, zucchini and tomatoes	60	
Brown rice (½ cup)	100	
Large tossed green salad w 1½ Tbsp low-cal dressing*	70	
Fresh fruit in season (apple, peach, etc)	70	
Water	0	515 Cal
* See page 40.		
SNACK		
Fiber One Chocolate Fudge Brownie	90	
Skim milk (4 oz)	40	130 Cal
		1200 Cal

Day 2 – 1200 Calorie Meal Plan

BREAKFAST	Calories	Totals
Orange juice (½ cup)	50	
Soft-boiled egg	80	
Whole-grain toast (1 slice) (Notes - page 42)	65	
Coffee	10	205 Cal
SNACK		
Coffee or tea	10	10 Cal
LUNCH		
Salad (3 oz tuna, 1 tsp Evoo, onions & celery)	175	
Lettuce & tomato wedges	20	
Rye bread (1 slice)	70	
Fresh fruit in season (pear, peach, etc)	70	
Coffee or tea	10	345 Cal
SNACK		
Yogurt (6 oz, nonfat, any flavor)	90	
Coffee or tea	10	100 Cal
DINNER		
Portobello burger (Day 2 Recipe- page 26)	270	
Lettuce and sliced tomato	20	
Whole-grain hard roll	140	
Steamed green beans	25	
Pickle spear	0	
Water	0	465 Cal
SNACK		
One small cookie	80	
Coffee or tea	10	90 Cal
		1205 Cal

Day 3 – 1200 Calorie Meal Plan

BREAKFAST	Calories	Totals
Orange juice (½ cup)	50	
Two blueberry pancakes (Day 3a Recipe- p.27)	190	
Light syrup (1½ Tbsp)	45	
Coffee	10	365 Cal
*Max of 30 Cal per Tbsp.		
SNACK		
Coffee or tea	10	10 Cal
LUNCH		
Peanut butter (2 Tbsp) on 2 slices bread	330	
Skim milk (4 oz)	45	375 Cal
SNACK		
Coffee or tea	10	10 Cal
DINNER		
Eggplant Parmesan (Day 3b Recipe- page 28)	270	
Large tossed salad w 1½ Tbsp low-cal dressing	70	
Italian or French bread (1 slice)	80	
Water	0	430 Cal
SNACK		
Coffee or tea	10	10 Cal
		1200 Cal

Day 4 – 1200 Calorie Meal Plan

BREAKFAST	Calories	Totals
Cantaloupe (½ medium)	50	
Fried egg	80	
Toasted raisin bread (1 slice)	75	
Coffee	10	215 Cal
SNACK		
Coffee or tea	10	10 Cal
LUNCH		
Soup #4 (Appendix C - page 42)*	180	
Lettuce & tomato sandwich (1 Tbsp light mayo)	170	
Cucumber slices and carrot & celery sticks	15	
Hot or iced tea	10	375 Cal
* Enjoy entire can (2 servings)		
SNACK		
Yogurt (6 oz, nonfat, any flavor)	90	
Coffee or tea	10	100 Cal
DINNER		
Tofu Veggie Stir Fry (Day 4 Recipe - page 29)	230	
Whole-grain bread (1 slice)	70	
Fresh fruit in season (apple, peach, etc)	70	
Water with lemon section	10	380 Cal
SNACK		
Popcorn Mini Bag	110	
Coffee or tea	10	120 Cal
		1200Cal

Day 5 – 1200 Calorie Meal Plan

BREAKFAST	Calories	Totals
Orange juice (½ cup)	50	
Cheerios (1 cup) + ½ cup skim milk	160	
Coffee	10	220 Cal
SNACK		
Yogurt (6 oz, nonfat, any flavor)	90	
Coffee or tea	10	100 Cal
LUNCH		
Soup #8 (Appendix C - page 42)	160	
Tomato slices, ¼ cup chopped basil + ½ tsp Evoo	40	
Whole-grain bread (1 slice)	65	
Hot or iced tea	10	275 Cal
SNACK		
Coffee or tea	10	10 Cal
DINNER		
Frozen vegetarian entree (Day 5 Recipe page 30)	300	
Large tossed green salad w 1½ Tbsp low-cal dressing	70	
Fresh fruit in season (peach, plum, etc)	70	
Water with lemon section	10	450 Cal
SNACK		
Two small cookies*	150	
Coffee or tea	10	160 Cal
* Check calories!		
		1215 Cal

Day 6 – 1200 Calorie Meal Plan

BREAKFAST	Calories	Totals
Orange juice (½ cup)	50	
Fried egg	80	
Whole-grain toast (1 slice)	65	
Coffee	10	205 Cal
SNACK		
Yogurt (6 oz, nonfat, any flavor)	90	
Coffee or tea	10	100 Cal
LUNCH		
Grilled Swiss cheese sandwich (2 oz low-fat	310	
Pickle spear	0	
Hot or iced tea	10	320 Cal
SNACK		
Fresh fruit in season (apple, plum, etc)	70	
Coffee or tea	10	80 Cal
DINNER		
Baked Herb-Crusted Cod (Day 6 Recipe page 31)	230	
Asparagus (7 spears cooked & drained)	20	
Large tossed green salad w 1½ Tbsp low-cal dressing	70	
Water with lemon section	15	335 Cal
SNACK		
Dark chocolate (1 oz)	150	
Coffee or tea	10	160 Cal
		1200 Cal

Day 7 – 1200 Calorie Meal Plan

BREAKFAST	Calories	Totals
Orange juice (½ cup)	50	
Shredded Wheat (1 cup) + ½ cup milk + ½ banana	260	
Coffee	10	320 Cal
SNACK		
Coffee or tea	10	10 Cal
LUNCH		
Egg salad (1 egg + 1 Tbsp light mayo)	125	
Small whole-grain roll	80	
Hot or iced tea	10	315 Cal
SNACK		
Coffee or tea	10	10 Cal
DINNER		
Pasta w Marinara sauce (Day 7 Recipe page 32)	225	
Large green salad with 1½ Tbsp low-cal dressing	70	
Fresh fruit in season (pear, plum, etc)	70	
Italian or French bread (1 slice)	80	
Water with lemon section	15	460 Cal
SNACK		
Fiber One Chocolate Fudge Brownie	90	
Coffee or tea	10	100 Cal
		1215 Cal

Recipes & Diet Tips

24

Day 1 Recipe

<u>Baked Salmon with Salsa</u>

This is a simple, straight-forward recipe. The advantage of a simple recipe is that there are no hidden calories.

> 4 - 5 oz salmon fillets
>
> 6 - Tbsp bottled tomato-pepper salsa

Brown salmon fillets in non-stick pan and place in baking dish. Put fillets in an oven preheated to 350 °F for about 10 minutes. Plate the salmon. Stir prepared tomato-pepper salsa and spoon it over the salmon.

<u>Serves 4</u>. One salmon fillet is about 215 Calories.

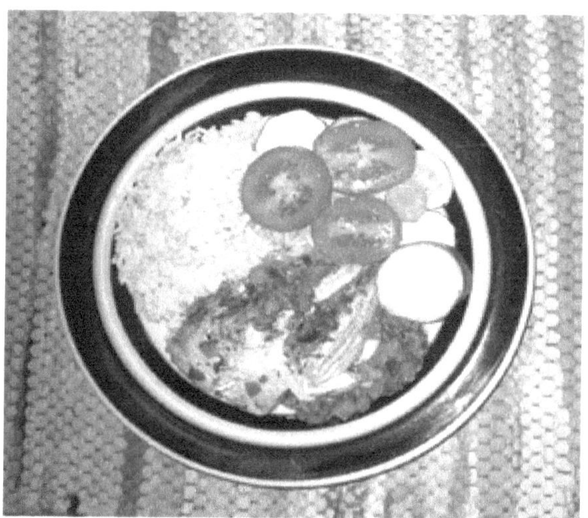

<u>Diet Tip of the Day:</u> **Have soup more often.** Most <u>non-cream-based</u> soups are filling and low-calorie.

Day 2 Recipe

<u>Portobello Mushroom Burger</u>

- ¼ cup low-sodium soy sauce
- ¼ cup balsamic vinegar
- 2 tablespoons olive oil
- 3 garlic cloves, minced
- 4 (4-inch) portobello mushroom caps
- 1 small red bell pepper
- ¼ cup light mayonnaise
- ½ teaspoon olive oil
- ⅛ teaspoon ground red pepper
- 4 (2-ounce) sandwich buns
- 4 (¼-inch-thick) slices tomato
- 4 curly leaf lettuce leaves

1. Combine first 4 ingredients in a large zip-top plastic bag; add mushrooms to bag. Seal and marinate at room temperature for 2 hours, turning bag occasionally. Remove mushrooms from bag. Start grill to medium heat.

3. Cut bell pepper in half lengthwise; discard seeds and membranes. Place pepper halves on grill rack coated with cooking spray; grill 15 minutes or until blackened, turning occasionally. Place in a zip-top plastic bag; seal. Let stand 10 minutes. Peel. Finely chop 1 pepper half; place in a small bowl. Add mayonnaise, ½ teaspoon oil, and ground red pepper; stir well.

4. Place mushrooms, gill sides down, on grill rack coated with cooking spray; grill 4 minutes on each side. Place buns, cut sides down, on grill rack coated with cooking spray; grill 30 seconds on each side or until toasted. Spread 2 tablespoons mayonnaise mixture on top half of each bun. Place 1 mushroom on bottom half of each bun. Top each mushroom with 1 tomato slice and 1 lettuce leaf.

<u>Serves 4</u>. About 270 Calories per serving.

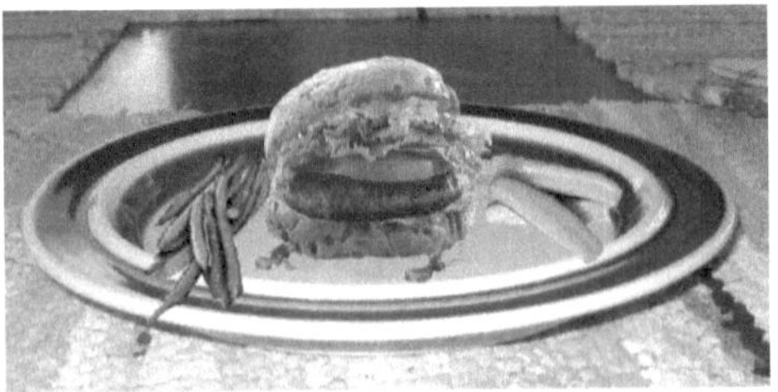

<u>Diet Tip of the Day:</u> **Drink lots of water** – about 8 glasses per day. Often, when you think you're hungry, you are just thirsty. So, next time you need a snack, drink some water and see if that does it for you.

26

<h1 style="text-align:center">Day 3a Recipe</h1>

Wild Blueberry Pancakes

This recipe makes a relatively low calorie, wholesome batch of delicious wild blueberry-whole wheat-buttermilk pancakes.

    1 cup whole-wheat flour
    1 cup buttermilk
    1 egg
    1 tablespoon vegetable oil
    1 teaspoon baking powder
    ½ teaspoon baking soda

Stir ingredients until blended. Add ¾ cup fresh of frozen blueberries and gently stir. Using medium heat, preheat a non-stick skillet coated with cooking spray. Pour slightly less than ¼ cup of batter onto skillet per pancake. Cook slowly until bubbles break on surface of pancake. Turn and cook until other side is lightly browned.

Makes 8 pancakes. Pictured below are three wild-blueberry pancakes with a special blueberry syrup. Sorry only two pancakes and light syrup are allowed on the 900 and 1200 Calorie diets.

Serves 4. Each pancake is about 95 Calories

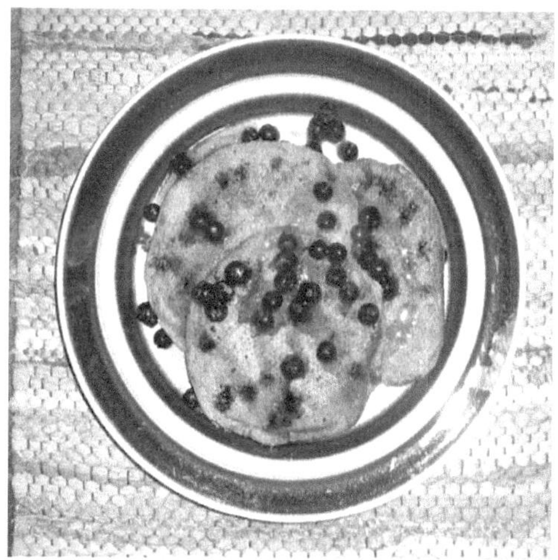

Three pancakes only allowed on 1500 Calorie diet.

Diet Tip of the Day: Most experts associate eating a substantial breakfast with successful weight loss.

Day 3b Recipe

Lo-Cal Eggplant Parmesan

   3 medium eggplants, cut crosswise into ½-inch slices
   3 tablespoons olive oil
   1 large onion, finely chopped
   1 large clove garlic, thinly sliced
   1½ teaspoons dried oregano
   1 28-ounce can no-salt plum tomatoes or crushed tomatoes
   1 tablespoon red wine vinegar
   ½ cup (packed) fresh basil leaves
   ½ cup freshly grated Parmesan cheese
   ⅓ cup fine dry bread crumbs

1. Preheat oven to 450°F. Brush both sides of eggplant slices with olive oil, and place in a single layer on baking sheets. Bake until undersides are golden brown, 10 to 15 minutes, then turn and bake until other sides are lightly browned. Set aside. Reduce oven to 375°F.

2. Meanwhile, in a large saucepan over medium heat, add 2 tablespoons olive oil, onion, oregano and garlic. Sauté until soft, about 10 minutes. Add plum tomatoes and their juices. Break up whole tomatoes. Cover, reduce heat to low and simmer 15 to 20 minutes.

3. Add vinegar, basil and salt and pepper to taste. In a 10-by-6-inch baking pan, spoon a small amount of tomato sauce, then add a thin scattering of parmesan cheese, then a single layer of eggplant. Repeat until all ingredients are used, ending with a little sauce and a sprinkling of parmesan cheese. In a small bowl, combine bread crumbs with enough olive oil to moisten. Sprinkle on top.

4. Bake until eggplant mixture is bubbly and center is hot, 30 to 45 minutes depending on size of pan and thickness of layers. Remove from heat and allow to rest before serving.

Serves 5.   About 270 Calories per serving

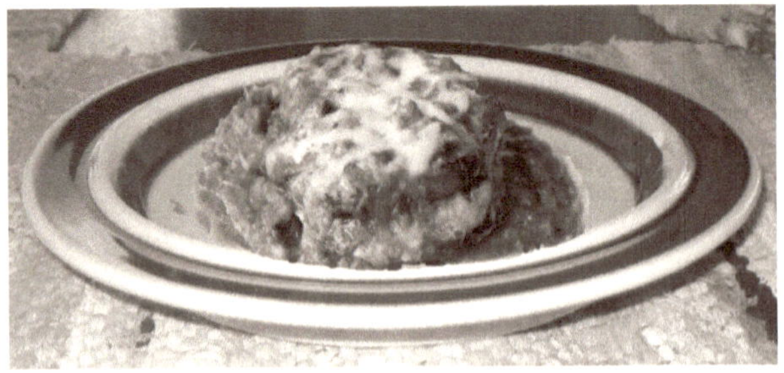

Diet Tip of the Day: If you find yourself at a party, don't stand near the food! Be aware of the temptation. Make the effort, and you'll find you eat less.

Day 4 Recipe

<u>Tofu-Veggie Stir Fry</u>

Citrus Sauce:

 6 tablespoons cooking wine
 ¼ cup orange juice
 1 tablespoon light soy sauce
 2 teaspoons toasted sesame oil
 1 teaspoon grated or minced fresh ginger
 1 teaspoon cornstarch
 1 tablespoon toasted sesame seeds

Stir Fry:

 1 (14-ounce) package firm tofu, drained
 1 tablespoon cooking oil
 1½ cups fresh or frozen sugar snap peas
 3 medium carrots, thinly sliced
 ¾ cup thinly sliced onion

1. Stir together sauce ingredients. Set aside while preparing stir fry.
2. Press and pat tofu dry with a towel to remove excess water. Cut into ½-inch cubes.
3. Heat a large skillet or wok over medium-high heat. Add oil and tofu; stir frequently until tofu is lightly browned, about 5 minutes. Add snow peas, carrots and onion. Stir-fry about 5 minutes until vegetables are cooked, but still crisp.
4. Stir in prepared sauce and cook 1-2 minutes until sauce is slightly thickened. Serve immediately.

<u>**Serves 4.**</u> 230 Calories per serving

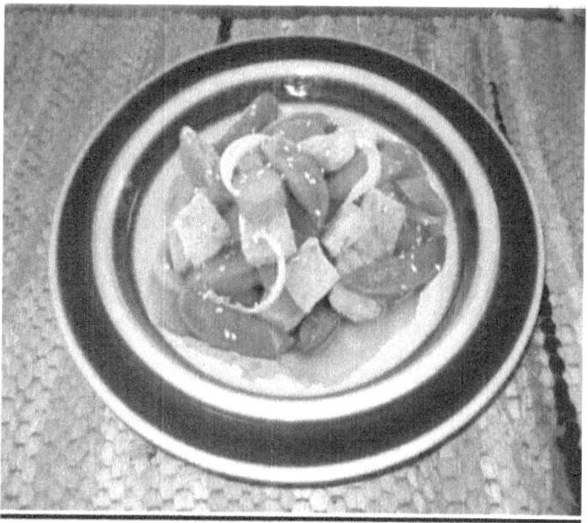

<u>**Diet Tip of the Day:**</u> Hot or cold cereal topped with fruit, and fat-free milk makes a nutritious, relatively low-calorie meal anytime.

Day 5 Recipe

<u>Frozen Vegetarian Dinner</u>

No recipe today. No cooking today. It's your day off! Some reasonably good frozen vegetarian dinners are:
- Amy's Indian Vegetable Korma (310 Cal)
- Amy's Thai Stir Fry (310 Cal)
- Amy's Asian Noodle Stir Fry (300 Cal)
- Lean Cuisine Veggie Scramble (180 Cal)
- Lean Cuisine Mushroom & Spring Pea Risotto (240 Cal)
- Healthy Choice Asian Potstickers (330 Cal)

The calorie allotment for the frozen entree are:
- 900-Calorie diet: 240 Calories
- 1200-Calorie diet: 340 Calories
- 1500-Calorie diet: 340 Calories

If you do not use all the calories allotted for this meal, use the excess calories anyway you wish. Splurge on extra dessert or save the calories for another day!

<u>Diet Tip of the Day:</u> Buy a pedometer and start walking. For the average person 2,100 steps amounts to walking about one mile. A Harvard study has shown that 8,000 to 10,000 step per day promote weight loss. And you're not obliged to walk continuously until you accrue all 10,000 steps. Rather, all steps throughout the day to wherever and whenever count toward your daily total. Because 10,000 steps a day may not be achievable by some people, particularly those who are elderly, sedentary, or who have chronic diseases, rather than insisting on a blanket 10,000 steps per day, your initial stepping goal should your baseline steps plus an increment of an additional 2,500 steps . (Your baseline being the number of steps you take in an average day.)

Day 6 Recipe

<u>Baked Herb-Crusted Cod</u>

      4 - 4 to 5 ounce cod fish fillets
      2 - tablespoons (Tbsp) flour
      2 - Tbsp cornmeal
      2 - Tbsp minced fresh herbs
      2 - teaspoons (tsp) lemon juice

Sprinkle cod with lemon juice. Mix flour, cornmeal and herbs and dust the cod with the cornmeal- herb mixture. Bake in oven at 375 °F for 10 minutes. Add salt and black pepper to taste.

<u>Serves 4</u>. One serving is about 230 Calories (for cod only).

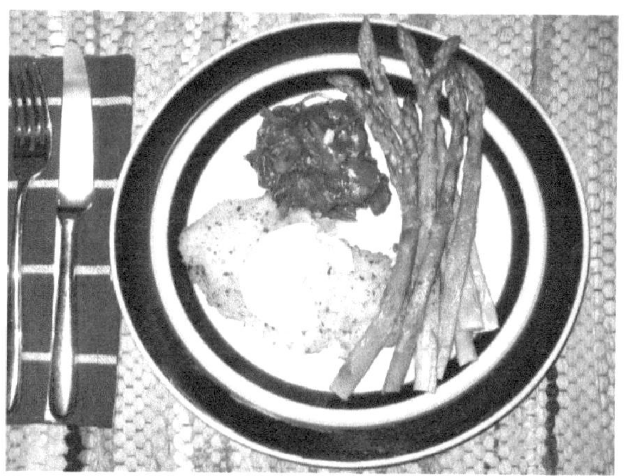

<u>Diet Tip of the Day:</u> **Take a daily multi-vitamin/mineral supplement.**
This is important when you're on a diet – as a kind of insurance policy.

31

Day 7 Recipe

Pasta with Marinara Sauce

Tomato sauce: Sauté ½ small onion, chopped fine, in 1 tsp olive oil. Add two finely chopped garlic cloves, 1½ cups chopped plum tomatoes and ½ tsp chopped fresh oregano. Stir and cook about 5 minutes on a low flame. (Later add about ¼ cup of the pasta liquid to the sauce to thin it.)

    ½ pound <u>whole-wheat</u> pasta

    ¼ tsp salt

Bring 2 quarts of lightly salted water to a boil. Add pasta and stir occasionally (to keep pasta from sticking to the bottom of the pot). Keep water boiling and cook until pasta are "al dente." (Cooking time is approximately 9 minutes.) Drain pasta. (Remember to add some of the pasta liquid to the tomato sauce.). Pour the marinara sauce over the pasta and serve hot.

<u>Serves 4</u>. One serving is about 225 Calories.

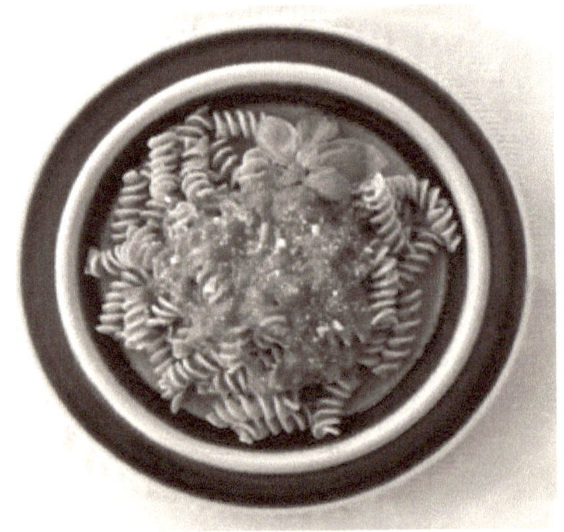

<u>Diet Tip of the Day:</u> **Beware of alcoholic beverages.** Beer has about 13 Calories per ounce, wine 25 Calories per ounce and whiskey 71 Calories per ounce.

Appendix A
Vegetarian Info

People choose a vegetarian, or plant-based diet, for reasons of nutrition, health, taste, morality, religion, culture, ethics, aesthetics, environment, economy, or politics.

Vegetarian Benefits

Compared to meat eaters, vegetarians have a lower overall mortality rate and a reduced incidence of heart disease, type 2 diabetes and stroke. And a vegetarian diet has been shown to reduce the risk of some cancers.

Properly planned vegetarian diets have been found to satisfy nutritional needs for all stages of life. Such diets have lower levels of saturated fat and cholesterol and higher levels of carbohydrates, fiber, magnesium, potassium, folate and antioxidants such as vitamins C and E and phytochemicals. And most nutritionists agree that properly planned vegetarian diets are nutritionally adequate and provide health benefits in the prevention and treatment of certain diseases. Large-scale studies have shown vegetarian diets significantly lower the risk of colon cancer, heart disease, high blood pressure and other diseases. In fact, many health-care professionals think that <u>eating a healthy vegetarian diet</u> is one of the best things you can do for your short-term and long-term health. In fact, a well planned vegetarian diet provides the same level of nutrients as a meat-eater's diet.

On the other hand, poorly planned vegetarian diets can increase the risk of cardiovascular disease, blood clots and platelet disorders. (These risks can be offset by sufficient consumption of vitamin B_{12} and polyunsaturated fatty acids.)

Vegetarian Nutrition

Vegetarian, or not, you should always consider the health effects of what you eat. Be sure to replace meat with healthy foods and eat a balanced diet. Eat a variety of whole grains, vegetables and protein foods, such as tofu or veggie burgers to stay full and healthy. While eating an adequate amount of protein is important for vegetarians, getting sufficient calcium and iron (and if you are a vegan vitamin B_{12}) are equally important.

The problem with some vegetarian diets is that they are often relatively low in omega-3 fatty acids and vitamin B_{12}. Conversely, high levels of dietary fiber, folic acid, vitamins C and E, and magnesium, and low consumption of saturated fat are all beneficial aspects of a vegetarian diet.

A well-balanced vegetarian diet with plenty of whole grains, fruits and vegetables is one of the healthiest diets on the planet. You do, however, need to make sure you get ample amounts of the following vital nutrients and micronutrients.

Protein
Most people eat too much protein – not too little of it. Adults need about 0.79 grams of protein for every kilogram of body weight per day to keep from slowly breaking down their own tissue. (That translates as approximately 0.36 grams of protein for every pound of body weight.) A case in point, an adult female weighing 154 pounds (70 kg) requires about (154 x 0.36), or 55 grams of protein per day. An adult male weighing 180 pounds requires (180 x 0.36), or 65 grams per day. How much protein is in food? A few examples: There are approximately seven grams of protein per ounce of beef, poultry, fish, cheese or peanuts. Soybeans pack 10 grams of protein per ounce. Most other beans and lentils contain about six grams of protein per ounce. There are roughly three grams of protein in an ounce of whole-grain cereal, and milk has one gram of protein per fluid ounce.

One cup of tofu contains about 20 grams of protein. Lots of foods contain protein and if vegetarians eat a well-balanced diet, they should undoubtedly consume more than enough protein without even thinking about it. Lacto-ovo vegetarians get sufficient protein from eggs and dairy. Pescaterians get all the protein they need from sea food, eggs and dairy. While vegans can get their protein from tofu, veggie burgers, soy, lentils, chickpeas, nuts and seeds, brown rice and whole grains.

Proteins are composed of amino acids. Often a concern with vegetarian and non-vegetarian is adequate intake of the eight essential amino acids, which cannot be synthesized by humans. While dairy and egg products provide complete protein sources for ovo-lacto vegetarians, several vegetable foods such as, soy, lupin beans, pumpkin seeds, hempseed, chia seeds, amaranth, buckwheat, pistachio nuts, and quinoa, also have significant amounts of all eight types of essential amino acids. Essential amino acids, can also be obtained by eating complementary plant sources that, in combination, provide all eight essential amino acids (e.g. brown rice and beans, whole wheat pasta and beans, or hummus and whole wheat pita,- though combining these in the same meal is not necessary). Protein intake in vegetarian diets is often lower than in meat diets but usually meets the daily requirements of most people. Numerous studies confirm that vegetarian diets supply sufficient protein provided a variety of plant sources are consumed.

Iron

Vegetarian diets typically contain similar levels of iron to non-vegetarian diets, but the iron is often not absorbed as well as iron from meat sources. In

addition, iron absorption is sometimes inhibited by other foods in the diet. Some dieticians recommend consuming foods high in vitamin C, such as citrus fruit or juices, tomatoes, or broccoli, as a way to increase the amount of iron absorbed. Vegetarian foods that are rich in iron are black beans, kidney beans, broccoli, lentils, oatmeal, raisins, spinach, cabbage, lettuce, black-eyed peas, soybeans, many breakfast cereals, sunflower seeds, chickpeas, tomato juice, molasses, thyme, and whole-wheat bread. Vegan diets are often higher in iron than lacto-vegetarian diets, because dairy products are low in iron. The American Dietetic Association, asserts that iron deficiency is no more common in vegetarians than in meat eaters, and iron deficiency anemia is rare in all diets.

Vitamin B_{12}

Vitamin B_{12} is not generally found in plants but is occurs naturally in foods of animal origin. Lacto-ovo vegetarians can obtain vitamin B_{12} from dairy products and eggs, while vegans can obtain vitamin B_{12} from a dietary supplement and fortified foods (such as some soy products and breakfast cereals). The recommended dietary allowance for B_{12} in the United States is 2.4 mcg per day and 2.8 mcg per day for lactating females. Although the daily requirement for vitamin B_{12} is very small, a vitamin B_{12} deficiency is very serious and can lead to anemia and irreversible nerve damage.

Fatty Acids

Omega-3 and omega-6 fatty acids are called "essential" fats for good reason. Humans need them for many functions, from building healthy cells to maintaining brain and nerve function. But our bodies cannot produce them. The only source is food. These polyunsaturated fats are also important because they lower the risk of heart disease. Some studies suggest these fats may also protect against type 2 diabetes, Alzheimer's disease, and age-related brain decline.

Omega-6 comes from soybean oil, corn oil and sunflower oil, as well as from nuts and seeds. The American Heart Association recommends that at least 5% to 10% of daily food calories come from omega-6 fatty acids. Omega-3 comes primarily from fatty fish such as salmon, mackerel, and tuna, and in lesser amounts from walnuts and flaxseeds.

Calcium

Calcium intake in vegetarians and vegans can be similar to that in meat eaters, provided the diet is properly planned. Lacto-ovo vegetarians consume dairy products and can obtain calcium from dairy sources like milk, yogurt, and cheese. Non-dairy milks that are fortified with calcium, such as soymilk and almond milk also contribute a significant amount of calcium to the diet. The calcium found in broccoli, bok choy, and kale is also well absorbed by the body. Though the calcium content per serving is lower in these vegetables than in a glass of milk, the absorption of the calcium is higher. Other foods that contain calcium include calcium-set tofu, blackstrap molasses, turnip greens, mustard greens, soybeans, almonds, okra, and dried figs. Although calcium is found in spinach, Swiss chard, beans and beet greens, the calcium in these foods is poorly absorbed by humans.

Vitamin D

Vitamin D is found in many foods, including fish, eggs, fortified milk, and cod liver oil. In addition, 10 minutes of sensible daily sun exposure is sufficient to prevent vitamin D deficiency. Vitamin D comes in several different types. Two forms are important to humans: vitamin D2, which is made by plants, and vitamin D3, which is made by human skin when exposed to sunlight. Foods may also be fortified with vitamin D2 or D3. The major role of vitamin D is to maintain normal blood levels of calcium and phosphorus. Vitamin D helps the body absorb calcium, which forms and maintains strong bones. It is used alone or together with calcium to improve bone health and decrease fractures. Vitamin D is thought to also protect against osteoporosis, high blood pressure, cancer, and other diseases.

Tofu Info

Tofu is an excellent non-animal high-protein food made from soybeans that is frequently linked with vegetarianism. Tofu comes in two basic varieties: soft or silken tofu and firm or regular tofu. Tofu has no taste but readily absorbs the flavor of other foods. Refrigerate tofu after you open a package and use it within four days.

Firm versions of tofu (well-drained) are used for kebabs, mock meats, and dishes requiring a consistency that holds together, while the softer tofu styles are used in desserts, soups, shakes, and sauces. Grated firm western tofu is sometimes used as a meat substitute and can be barbecued because it will hold together on a barbecue grill. Soft tofu is sometimes used as a dairy-free or low-calorie filler. Silken tofu may be used to replace cheese in certain dishes such as lasagna.

Most proteins are delicious even when seasoned simply with salt and pepper. Not tofu which most often tofu tastes bland. But you can turn it into a food you actually want to eat with the following tips.

Buying Tofu

Tofu is usually found in a refrigerated case in the produce department (fruit and vegetables) of most supermarkets. Some stores have tofu in the dairy section and others in stock it in health-food.

Preparing Tofu

1) Most tofu comes packed in water. But a water-logged block of tofu won't absorb a marinade or get crispy in a frying pan. The first thing to do is drain the block as much as possible. To drain it, slice the block and place the slices on a paper towel-lined baking sheet. Top tofu with more paper towels and then a heavy object. Let tofu sit at least one hour. Once drained, you can marinate the tofu or start cooking it.

2) After pressing, tofu is ready to absorb flavor. But the tofu still retains some water and oil and water don't mix. In most cases, use soy, citrus, or vinegar-based marinades instead.

3) Trying to get tofu crispy is difficult. Tossing tofu in cornstarch overcomes the difficulty. Place cornstarch in a bowl, add drained or marinated tofu pieces, and toss. A light coating is best.

4) To sear tofu, use sesame oil which can take the heat and doubles as a flavoring agent, giving the tofu a nutty flavor.

Leftover Tofu

Once a package of tofu is opened it will last about three days if refrigerated. You can freeze leftover tofu. Frozen tofu can last up to three months. And you can freeze any kind of tofu: silken, firm, or extra firm. Just cut the tofu into cubes and freeze the cubes on a baking sheet. Once hard, store the tofu together in a freezer container. Thaw leftover tofu on a counter top during dinner prep. Thawed tofu can be cooked just as fresh tofu. But squeeze the tofu gently before cooking to eliminate extra moisture.

Appendix B
Eat Smart

Every good weight-loss diet must have the following three characteristics: **First**, a good diet must provide you with an understanding of weight control as well as the knowledge you need to reduce your weight to the desired level. **Second**, a good diet must help you remain healthy while you are losing weight. **Third**, a good diet must lead you to a healthier way of eating and exercising that will, in the long term, help you keep off the weight you have lost.

The weight-loss diet featured in this eBook is the so-called "balanced diet;" i.e., a diet that is not only low calorie and reasonably low in fat, but is also nutritionally balanced. The *7-Day Diet for women*, however, does not meet all the criteria set forth above. While you will get some "dieting insight" and some idea of how much you can eat and still lose weight, you will not get a real understanding of weight control from this eBook. That's not its purpose. What you will get is a healthy diet – and a diet that if followed will promote weight loss. Think of the *7-Day Diet* as a quick fix, a healthy start that will get you on the right track – but it's not the long-term answer.

Long-term success is about developing both an understanding and a plan that will result in healthier eating and physical activity habits. The desire to lose weight and the discipline to start and stay on a weight-control program are crucial. But along with desire and discipline, it is our belief that **only an in-depth understanding of weight control, nutrition and exercise will lead to long-term success**. For a through understanding and the guidance you need to succeed in the long term I recommend you read, *Weight Control - U.S. Edition* by Vincent Antonetti, Ph.D., an eBook also published by NoPaperPress.

Breakfast Guidelines

You've heard it before. It's important to start the day right and eat breakfast. **So try to allow time for breakfast before you rush off to work.** If need be do some preliminary preparation the night before such as setting up your coffee maker, deciding on and measuring the amount of cereal you will be eating, etc. Many busy people prepare breakfast at home and bring it to work in a plastic container. Do what you need to do – but don't skip breakfast!

In the *7-Day Vegetarian Diet,* you may substitute wholesome **whole-grain cereal** for any specified cereal. For example, if you're not crazy about having Shredded Wheat for breakfast on Day 6, substitute Wheat Chex or Cheerios, etc. And if you don't like the fried egg called for on Day 5, have a hard-boiled egg or make a scrambled egg instead. Maybe the cantaloupe called for in the meal plan is not in season. No problem. Just replace the cantaloupe with a half cup of orange juice.

Lunch Guidelines

On most days of the *7-Day Diet,* lunch will call for either soup or a sandwich. Feel free to substitute a soup you favor in place of those indicated – provided the basic type of soup and calorie counts are similar to those specified in the *7-Day Diet.* For example, Day 1 calls for a cup of Lentil Soup (140 Calories), but if you prefer, you may substitute a cup of Navy Bean Soup – which is in the same food group as lentil soup and contains approximately the same calorie count.

Warm Weather Substitutions: On warm and especially very hot days, you may want to substitute a sandwich, a tuna or salmon salad for the soup of the day.

Dinner Guidelines

On the *7-Day Diet Vegetarian*, one of the dinner mainstays is a "Tossed Green Salad." Prepare your "Tossed Green Salad" in a bowl with a volume of at least 16 ounces, or 2 cups. First add about 1 cup of either green leaf lettuce, Romaine lettuce or a mesclun mix. Then add, as desired, half cup of green veggies such as broccoli, celery, cucumber, peppers, spinach, or watercress. This vegetable combination will, on average, total about 35 Calories. You will be eating a "Tossed Green Salad" just about every day at dinnertime. Remember that variety is the key to a nutritious diet. So be sure to vary the ingredients of the salad.

Top your "Tossed Green Salad" with 2 tablespoons of any light salad dressing available at your local supermarket that contains no more than 20 to 25 Calories per tablespoon. Some of my favorite light salad dressings are:
- **Kraft Light Done Right House Italian**
- **Wishbone Just 2 Good Honey Dijon**
- **Newman's Lighten Up! Balsamic Vinaigrette**

Your "Tossed Green Salad" with salad dressing will cost you roughly 70 Calories but will be packed with lots of health-giving vitamins, minerals and fiber.

Snack Guidelines

On some of the menus in the *7-Day Diet Vegetarian* feature a morning snack, an afternoon snack and an evening snack. The main snacks are:

Yogurt: We recommend Dannon Light at 90 Calories per container (at this writing). Select any flavor. There are other brands you may prefer but whatever you buy be certain you eat no more than 90 Calories worth of yogurt for your snack.

Fresh Fruit in season: Choose an apple, pear, peach, plum, watermelon (1 cup), etc. You will be eating fruit every day. So vary the fruit that you select to get good array of micronutrients.

Handful of Unsalted Mixed Nuts: Nuts and seeds are loaded with protein and fiber. This eBook uses a "handful" as a convenient descriptor rather than something like "16 almonds = 100 Calories," but be aware that although nuts are a healthy food, nuts are also a high-calorie food. Buy mixed nuts to get a range of micronutrients. And please no salt.

Skinny Cow Ice Cream Sandwich: This is a relatively low-calorie, low fat, yummy dairy-sweet snack.

Kashi TLC Chewy Granola Bar: A sweet treat packed with whole grains, nuts and seeds. The bar comes in four flavors – with each containing about 140 Calories.

Popcorn: Popcorn is a tasty, nutritious high-fiber, filling snack. A Popcorn Mini Bag, such as Orville Redenbacher's Smart Pop is convenient and contains 110 Calories. But for the best popcorn I suggest you purchase a hot-air popper which uses popping corn, a type of corn that bursts from the kernel and puffs up when heated. A hot-air popper will make a large batch of popcorn in a few minutes. For a snack, eat only 5 or 6 cups of the popcorn and store the remainder for another day. At this writing, you can buy a hot-air popper for approximately $25.00.

About Bread

First understand that bread, more specifically whole-grain breads, are good sources of complex carbohydrates and dietary fiber, as well as several B vitamins (thiamin, riboflavin, niacin, and folate), vitamin E, and minerals (iron, magnesium and selenium).

In recent years, however, sliced bread loaves have gotten larger, as have the bread slices inside these loaves. Just a few years ago the standard slice of bread contained about 70 Calories – now most are 100 plus Calories.

The *7-Day Diet* requires whole-grain bread at 70 Calories per slice. Quite a few bakers sell thin sliced or "light" sliced bread. The difficult part is finding a whole grain thin sliced or "light" bread (with about 70 Calories per slice). Whatever the brand, make sure the first word in the Ingredients list is "whole." "Pepperidge Farm Small Slice 100% Whole Wheat" is a good choice. It's whole grain, has 70 Calories per slice and it tastes good too.

Important Notes

1) If desired, skim milk and a sugar substitute may be added to coffee or tea. And soy or almond milk may be used instead of cow's milk.

2) Fried eggs, scrambled eggs, or an omelet should be cooked in a pan coated with a non-stick cooking spray.

3) On bread, corn on the cob and baked potatoes, if desired, you may use a zero-calorie butter substitute spray. Do not use butter!

4) Cereals should be whole grain and preferably without added sugar. At the top of the list are Old-fashioned Oat Meal, Wheatena and Shredded Wheat. Among other reasonably healthy choices are Cheerios, Wheat Chex, Wheaties, some Kashi cereals and Farina.

5) Bread may be either plain or toasted whole grain, such as whole wheat, whole rye or pumpernickel. If desired, bread may be sprayed with a zero-calorie butter substitute.

6) Use only lean cuts of meat trimmed of all visible fat. Poultry should be limited to chicken or turkey breasts (white meat only and skinless). Make sure the turkey bacon you use contains no more than 35 Calories per slice.

7) When canned tuna or salmon is specified, use only fish packed in water.

8) An unlimited amount of green salad may be eaten, but the salad dressing should be as specified.

9) Use freely as desired: clear unsweetened coffee, clear unsweetened tea, water, seltzer, any diet soda, clear soups without fat, bouillon, and seasonings such as mustard, cinnamon, dill, herbs, red and black pepper, curry, vinegar, lemon juice and sections, and dill and sour pickles.

10) Any specified snack may be moved to any other part of the day, and/or combined with breakfast, lunch or dinner.

Appendix C
Vegetarian Soup*

The following lists soup selections that come in cans and microwavable bowls. See the important note at the end of list regarding serving size. Valid as of 08/20/20.

Soup Description	**Container**	**Calories**
Amy's Organic Chunky Vegetable	Canned	60
Amy's Organic Minestrone	Canned	90
Healthy Choice Cheese Tortellini	Microwaveable	90
Amy's Organic Split Pea	Canned	100
Amy's No Chicken Noodle	Canned	100
Amy's Organic Butternut Squash	Canned	100
Healthy Choice Country Vegetable	Microwaveable	100
Amy's Organic Vegan Chunky Tomato	Canned	110
Healthy Choice Red Bean and Rice	Microwaveable	130
Healthy Choice Tomato Basil	Microwaveable	130
Amy's Organic Southwestern Vegetable	Canned	140
Amy's Organic Hearty Spanish Rice &	Canned	140
Amy's Organic Hearty Rustic Italian	Canned	140
Amy's Organic Thai Coconut	Canned	140
Healthy Choice Vegetable Barley	Microwaveable	140
Amy's Organic Quinoa, Kale & Red	Canned	150
Healthy Choice Traditional Lentil	Microwaveable	160
Amy's Organic Lentil Vegetable	Canned	160
Amy's Indian Golden Lentil	Canned	220

* **Important:** When the Daily Meal Plan menu specifies soup, have only one serving (usually this is 1 cup = 8 ounces) unless stated otherwise.

NoPaperPress Paperbacks and eBooks

100-Day Super Diet-1200 Calorie*
100-Day Super Diet-1500 Calorie*
100-Day No-Cooking Diet-1200 Cal*
100-Day No-Cooking Diet-1500 Cal*
90-Day Smart Diet-1200 Calorie*
90-Day Smart Diet-1500 Calorie*
90-Day No-Cooking Diet - 1200 Cal*
90-Day No-Cooking Diet - 1500 Cal*
90-Day Perfect Diet - 1200 Calorie*
90-Day Perfect Diet - 1500 Calorie*
60-Day Perfect Diet-1200 Calorie*
60-Day Perfect Diet-1500 Calorie*
50-Day Flex Diet-1200 Calorie*
50-Day Flex Diet-1500 Calorie*
30-Day Quick Diet - for Women*
30-Day Quick Diet - for Men*
30-Day No-Cooking Diet*
30-Day Diet for Women - Metric*
30-Day Diet for Men - Metric*
25 Day Easy Diet-1200 Calorie*
25 Day Easy Diet-1500 Calorie*
25-Day No-Cooking Diet
10-Day Express Diet
10-Day No-Cooking Diet*
7-Day Diet for Women*
7-Day Diet for Men*
7-Day No-Cooking Diets*
90-Day Gluten-Free Diet-1200 Cal*
90-Day Gluten-Free Diet-1500 Cal*
30-Day Gluten-Free Quick Diet*
30-Day Gluten-Free No-Cooking Diet*
7-Day Diet for Women - Metric*
7-Day Diet for Men - Metric
7-Day Gluten-Free Express Diet*
7-Day Gluten-Free No-Cooking Diet*
90-Day Vegetarian Diet-1200 Calorie*
90-Day Vegetarian Diet-1500 Calorie*
30-Day Vegetarian Diet*
7-Day Vegetarian Diet*
Weight Loss for Women*
Weight Loss for Women - Metric
Weight Loss for Women - UK
Weight Loss for Men*
Maximum Weight Loss - 1200 Cal*
Maximum Weight Loss - 1500 Cal*

Weight Loss for Men - Metric*
Maximum Weight Loss- 1200 Calorie*
Maximum Weight Loss- 1500 Calorie*
Weight Control - U.S. Edition
Weight Control - Metric. Edition
Professional Weight Control Women - U.S.
Professional Weight Control Women - Metric
Professional Weight Control Men - U.S.
Professional Weight Control Men - Metric
Weight Maintenance - U.S. Edition*
Weight Maintenance - Metric. Edition*
Weight Maintenance - UK Edition
Weight Loss for Senior Men*
Weight Loss for Senior Women*
Eat Smart - U.S. Edition*
Eat Smart - Metric Edition
30-Day Mediterranean Diet
Exercise Smart - U.S. Edition*
Exercise Smart - Metric Edition
Exercise Smart - UK Edition*
Total Fitness - U.S. Edition
Total Fitness - Metric Edition
Total Fitness - UK Edition
Total Fitness for Women-U.S. Edition*
Total Fitness for Women - Metric
Total Fitness for Women - UK Edition
Total Fitness for Men - U.S. Edition*
Total Fitness for Men- Metric Edition*
Total Fitness for Men - UK Edition
Senior Fitness - U.S. Edition*
Senior Fitness - Metric Edition*
Senior Fitness - UK Edition*
Computer Diet - U.S. Edition*
Computer Diet - Metric Edition*
Reliable Weight Loss - U.S. Edition
101 Weight Loss Tips*
101 Healthy Eating Tips*
101 Lifelong Fitness Tips*
101 Weight Maintenance Tips
101 Weight Loss Recipes
101 Gluten-Free Weight Loss Recipes
101 Vegetarian Weight Loss Recipes*
30-Day Mediterranean Diet*
90-Day Mediterranean Diet - 1200 Cal*
90-Day Mediterranean Diet - 1500 Cal*

* These titles are available as both ebooks and paperbacks. Our ebooks are sold by Amazon, Apple, Google, Barnes & Noble and Kobo. But paperbacks are only sold by Amazon.

Disclaimer

This book offers general meal planning, nutrition and weight control information. It is not a medical manual and the author does not claim to be medically qualified. The material in this book is not intended to be a substitute for medical counseling. Everyone should have a medical checkup before beginning a weight loss program. Moreover, the physician conducting the medical exam should be made aware of and should approve the specific weight control program planned. Additionally, while the author and publisher have made every effort to ensure the accuracy of the information in this book, they make no representations or warranties regarding its accuracy or completeness . Further, neither the author nor publisher assume liability for any medical problems that might result from applying the methods in this book, or for any loss of profit, or any other commercial damages, including but not limited to special, incidental, consequential or other damages, and any such liability is hereby disclaimed.